I0781755

Proven Strategies to Boost Productivity and Time Management
Dedication
To everyone striving to make the most of their time and achieve their goals. This book is for you.
Acknowledgements
I extend my deepest gratitude to my family and friends for their unwavering support and encouragement. Special thanks to all the productivity experts and thought leaders who have inspired and informed this work. Lastly, to my readers—thank you for taking the first step towards mastering your day and transforming your life.

Introduction

In today's fast-paced world, mastering productivity and time management is essential for success. Whether you're a student, a professional, or an entrepreneur, the ability to effectively manage your time can make the difference between achieving your goals and falling short. This book aims to provide you with proven strategies and practical tips to boost your productivity and make the most out of each day.

Table of Contents

Chapter 4: Overcoming Procrastination
Identifying the root causes of procrastination.
Practical strategies to overcome procrastination.
Maintaining motivation and momentum.
Chapter 5: Creating a Productive Environment
Setting up a workspace that minimizes distractions.
The role of the environment in enhancing productivity.
Tips for organizing physical and digital spaces.
Chapter 6: Utilizing Technology
Review of productivity apps and tools.
Balancing technology is used to avoid distractions.
Maximizing the benefits of digital tools.
Chapter 7: Work-Life Balance
Importance of maintaining a healthy work-life balance.
Strategies for setting boundaries and prioritizing self-care.
Tips for achieving balance between work and personal life.
Chapter 8: Continuous Improvement
Introduction to the concept of Kaizen (continuous improvement).
Regularly assessing and improving productivity routines.
Embracing a mindset of continuous learning and improvement.
Conclusion
Summarizing key points and strategies discussed in the book.
Encouragement to implement the strategies and stay committed to
the journey of productivity.
Final thoughts on making the most of your time to achieve a
balanced and fulfilling life.
Chapter 1: Understanding Productivity
What is Productivity?
Productivity is a measure of efficiency, specifically how effectively
you convert your time and energy into meaningful results. It's not
merely about completing as many tasks as possible, but about
prioritizing and executing tasks that align with your goals and
values. Productivity involves working smarter, not harder, to achieve
optimal results with minimal wasted effort.
Key Aspects of Productivity:
Efficiency: Completing tasks in the least amount of time without
compromising quality.
Effectiveness: Focusing on tasks that have the greatest impact on
your goals.

Prioritization: Identifying and addressing high-priority tasks first.
Consistency: Maintaining a steady pace of work over time.
Understanding the true essence of productivity requires a shift in mindset from being busy to being purposefully engaged in meaningful activities.

The Impact of Productivity on Success

High productivity levels can significantly influence both personal and professional success. When you are productive, you make the most of your available resources, including time, energy, and skills. This efficiency leads to a range of positive outcomes:

Personal Benefits:

Increased Satisfaction: Accomplishing your goals and seeing tangible progress boosts self-esteem and satisfaction.

Better Work-Life Balance: Efficiently managing your tasks frees up time for leisure, family, and self-care.

Reduced Stress : A structured approach to work can prevent last-minute rushes and reduce stress levels.

Professional Benefits:

Enhanced Performance: High productivity leads to better performance reviews, promotions, and career advancement.

Achievement of Goals: Effective task management helps you reach both short-term and long-term professional objectives.

Reputation Building : Being known as a productive and reliable individual can enhance your professional reputation and open up more opportunities.

By improving your productivity, you can achieve more in less time, paving the way for greater accomplishments and a more fulfilling life.

Common Misconceptions About Productivity

Many people have misconceptions about what it means to be productive. Dispelling these myths can help you adopt more effective productivity strategies.

Misconception 1: Productivity is About Doing More

One of the biggest misconceptions is that productivity is synonymous with doing more. In reality, productivity is about doing what matters most. It's about focusing on high-impact activities rather than filling your schedule with low-priority tasks.

Misconception 2: Multitasking Increases Productivity

Contrary to popular belief, multitasking often reduces productivity. Juggling multiple tasks can lead to mistakes and lower the quality of work. Focusing on one task at a time usually results in better outcomes.

Misconception 3: Longer Hours Mean Greater Productivity

Working longer hours doesn't necessarily equate to higher productivity. Overworking can lead to burnout and diminished returns. It's more effective to work smarter by taking breaks, setting boundaries, and ensuring you have time to recharge.

Misconception 4: Productivity is a Constant State

Productivity can fluctuate due to various factors such as energy levels, motivation, and external circumstances. Understanding that productivity has ebbs and flows allows you to be more compassionate with yourself and adjust your strategies accordingly.

Strategies for Enhancing Productivity

Now that we have a clear understanding of what productivity is and isn't, let's explore some effective strategies to enhance it.

1. Prioritize Tasks with the Eisenhower Matrix

Urgent and Important: Do these tasks immediately.

Important but Not Urgent: Schedule these tasks for later.

Urgent but Not Important: Delegate these tasks if possible.

Neither Urgent Nor Important: Eliminate these tasks.

2. Implement the Pomodoro Technique

Work for 25 minutes, then take a 5-minute break.

After four cycles, take a longer break (15-30 minutes).

This technique helps maintain focus and prevents burnout.

3. Set SMART Goals

Specific: Clearly define what you want to achieve.

Measurable: Determine how you will measure progress.

Achievable: Set realistic and attainable goals.

Relevant: Ensure your goals align with your broader objectives.

Time-bound: Set deadlines to keep yourself accountable.

4. Create a Productive Environment

Minimize distractions by organizing your workspace.

Use tools and apps to manage tasks and time effectively.

Establish routines that signal it's time to work.

5. Practice Mindfulness and Self-Care

Incorporate mindfulness practices like meditation to stay focused.

Ensure you are taking care of your physical health with proper nutrition, exercise, and sleep.

By applying these strategies, you can enhance your productivity and work more efficiently towards achieving your goals.

This chapter provides a foundational understanding of productivity, addressing its true nature, the impact it can have on success, common misconceptions, and practical strategies for improvement. The subsequent chapters will build on this foundation, offering more detailed techniques and insights to help you master your day and achieve your full potential.

Chapter 2: Setting Clear Goals

The Importance of Goal Setting

Setting clear goals is the cornerstone of productivity and success. Goals give direction and purpose to your actions, ensuring that your efforts are aligned with your desired outcomes. Without clear goals, it's easy to get sidetracked by less important tasks, leading to wasted time and energy.

Key Benefits of Goal Setting :

Focus: Goals help you concentrate your efforts on what truly matters.

Motivation: Clearly defined objectives provide a sense of purpose and drive.

Measurement: Goals allow you to track progress and measure success.

Accountability: Setting goals makes you accountable to yourself and others.

Goals act as a roadmap, guiding your decisions and actions towards achieving specific, meaningful outcomes.

How to Set SMART Goals

One of the most effective ways to set goals is by using the SMART criteria. SMART goals are:

Specific : Clearly define what you want to achieve. A specific goal has a much greater chance of being accomplished than a general one.

Example : Instead of "I want to get fit," a specific goal would be "I want to run a 5K marathon."

Measurable: Establish criteria for measuring progress. This allows you to track your progress and stay motivated.

Example : "I will track my running distance and time every week."

Achievable: Ensure that your goal is realistic and attainable. Setting overly ambitious goals can be discouraging.

Example : "I will increase my running distance by 1 mile every week."

Relevant: Your goal should matter to you and align with other relevant goals.

Example : "Running a 5K marathon will improve my overall health and fitness, which is important to me."

Time-bound: Set a deadline for your goal. This creates a sense of urgency and helps prevent procrastination.

Example : "I will complete my first 5K marathon within 3 months."

By setting SMART goals, you create a clear and actionable plan that increases your chances of success.

Breaking Down Long-Term Goals into Manageable Steps

Long-term goals can often seem overwhelming. Breaking them down into smaller, manageable steps makes them more achievable and helps maintain motivation.

Steps to Break Down Long-Term Goals:

Define the End Goal: Clearly articulate your long-term goal.

Example : "Run a marathon in a year."

Identify Milestones: Break the end goal into major milestones.

Example : "Run a 10K in three months, a half marathon in six months, and a full marathon in twelve months."

Create Action Plans for Each Milestone: Develop detailed plans for achieving each milestone.

Example:

Month 1: Run 3 miles three times a week.

Month 2: Increase to 5 miles three times a week.

Month 3: Run 10K (6.2 miles) race.

Set Weekly and Daily Goals: Further break down the action plans into weekly and daily goals.

Example:

Week 1: Run 2 miles on Monday, Wednesday, and Friday.

Week 2: Increase to 3 miles.

Review and Adjust: Regularly review your progress and adjust your plans as needed.

Example: If you miss a run, adjust the following week's plan to make up for it.

By breaking down long-term goals into smaller, more manageable steps, you create a clear path to success and make the process less daunting.

Staying Motivated and Overcoming Obstacles

Even with clear goals and a detailed plan, staying motivated and overcoming obstacles can be challenging. Here are some strategies to help you stay on track:

1. Visualize Success

Regularly visualize yourself achieving your goals. This can boost motivation and reinforce your commitment.

2. Reward Yourself

Set up a reward system for when you reach milestones. Rewards can be small, like treating yourself to a favorite snack, or larger, like taking a day off to relax.

3. Stay Flexible

Be prepared to adjust your goals and plans if needed. Life is unpredictable, and flexibility can help you stay on course even when things don't go as planned.

4. Seek Support

Share your goals with friends, family, or a mentor. Having a support system can provide encouragement and accountability.

5. Monitor Progress

Regularly check in on your progress and celebrate small wins. This helps maintain motivation and provides a sense of accomplishment.

6. Learn from Setbacks

Treat setbacks as learning opportunities. Analyze what went wrong, make necessary adjustments, and keep moving forward.

Staying motivated is crucial for achieving your goals, and these strategies can help you maintain your drive and overcome any obstacles you encounter along the way.

By setting clear, SMART goals and breaking them down into manageable steps, you lay a strong foundation for success. Staying motivated and flexible further enhances your ability to achieve these goals. In the next chapter, we will explore specific time management techniques that can help you effectively implement your goals and maximize your productivity.

Chapter 3: Time Management Techniques

Time management is essential for boosting productivity and achieving your goals. Effective time management helps you make the most out of each day, reduces stress, and increases your efficiency. This chapter explores various time management techniques that can help you stay organized and focused.

The Pomodoro Technique

The Pomodoro Technique is a popular time management method that involves breaking your work into short, focused intervals called "Pomodoros," followed by short breaks. This technique helps maintain high levels of concentration and prevents burnout.

How to Implement the Pomodoro Technique:

Choose a Task: Select a task you want to work on.

Set a Timer: Set a timer for 25 minutes. This period is called a Pomodoro.

Work on the Task: Focus solely on the task until the timer goes off. Avoid all distractions.

Take a Short Break: Once the timer goes off, take a 5-minute break. Use this time to relax, stretch, or grab a snack.

Repeat: After four Pomodoros, take a longer break (15-30 minutes) to rest and recharge.

Benefits of the Pomodoro Technique:

Enhanced Focus: Short, focused intervals help improve concentration.

Reduced Fatigue: Regular breaks prevent burnout and keep you energized.

Improved Productivity: Breaking tasks into manageable chunks makes them less daunting and easier to tackle.

The Eisenhower Matrix

The Eisenhower Matrix, also known as the Urgent-Important Matrix, helps you prioritize tasks based on their urgency and importance. This method ensures that you focus on tasks that truly matter and avoid getting bogged down by trivial ones.

How to Use the Eisenhower Matrix:

Draw a Grid: Divide a page into four quadrants.

Label the Quadrants:

Quadrant 1: Urgent and Important

Quadrant 2: Important but Not Urgent

Quadrant 3: Urgent but Not Important

Quadrant 4: Neither Urgent nor Important

Categorize Your Tasks: List your tasks in the appropriate quadrant.

Quadrant Analysis:

Quadrant 1 (Do First): Tasks that are both urgent and important. These tasks require immediate attention.

Example: Meeting deadlines, urgent problems.

Quadrant 2 (Schedule): Tasks that are important but not urgent. Schedule time to work on these tasks to prevent them from becoming urgent.

Example: Long-term projects, personal development.

Quadrant 3 (Delegate): Tasks that are urgent but not important. Delegate these tasks if possible.

Example: Interruptions, some emails.

Quadrant 4 (Eliminate): Tasks that are neither urgent nor important. These tasks are distractions and should be minimized or eliminated.

Example : Browsing social media, trivial activities.

Benefits of the Eisenhower Matrix:

Prioritization: Helps you identify and focus on tasks that matter most.

Efficiency: Reduces time spent on less important tasks.

Stress Reduction : Prevents last-minute rushes by addressing important tasks before they become urgent.

Time Blocking

Time blocking involves scheduling specific blocks of time for different tasks or activities throughout your day. This method helps you allocate dedicated time to important tasks, ensuring that they receive the attention they deserve.

How to Implement Time Blocking:

Identify Your Tasks: List all the tasks you need to complete.

Allocate Time Blocks: Assign specific time blocks for each task. Be realistic about how long each task will take.

Create a Schedule: Use a planner or digital calendar to block out time for each task.

Stick to the Schedule: Follow your time blocks as closely as possible. Avoid multitasking and stick to the task at hand during each block.

Benefits of Time Blocking:

Structured Day: Provides a clear plan for your day, reducing decision fatigue.

Increased Focus: Dedicated time blocks help you concentrate on one task at a time.

Better Time Management: Ensures that all important tasks receive attention.

Additional Time Management Techniques

1. The Two-Minute Rule

If a task takes less than two minutes to complete, do it immediately. This prevents small tasks from piling up and becoming overwhelming.

2. Batching Similar Tasks

Group similar tasks together and complete them in one session. For example, answer all emails at once instead of sporadically throughout the day. This reduces the cognitive load of switching between different types of tasks.

3. Setting Priorities with the ABCDE Method

Assign each task a priority level:

A: Must-do tasks with serious consequences if not completed.

B: Should-do tasks with mild consequences if not completed.

C: Nice-to-do tasks with no consequences if not completed.

D: Delegate tasks that can be done by someone else.

E: Eliminate tasks that are unnecessary.

Tackle A-level tasks first, then move to B-level tasks, and so on.

4. Using Technology for Time Management

Apps and Tools: Utilize productivity apps like Trello, Asana, or Todoist to manage tasks and projects.

Calendars: Digital calendars like Google Calendar can help you schedule and remind you of important tasks and deadlines.

Conclusion

Mastering time management is crucial for increasing productivity and achieving your goals. The Pomodoro Technique, Eisenhower Matrix, and Time Blocking are powerful methods that can help you manage your time more effectively. By implementing these techniques, you can focus on what truly matters, reduce stress, and make the most out of each day.

In the next chapter, we will explore how to overcome procrastination, a common barrier to effective time management and productivity. You will learn practical strategies to beat procrastination and maintain momentum towards achieving your goals.

Chapter 4: Overcoming Procrastination

Procrastination is a common challenge that many people face when trying to manage their time effectively. It involves delaying or avoiding tasks, often due to feelings of anxiety, fear, or lack of motivation. Overcoming procrastination is essential for maximizing productivity and achieving your goals. This chapter explores the root causes of procrastination and offers practical strategies to overcome it.

Understanding Procrastination

Procrastination is often fueled by various factors, including:

Fear of Failure:

The fear of not meeting expectations or making mistakes can paralyze individuals, leading them to avoid tasks altogether.

Perfectionism:

Striving for perfection can be a double-edged sword. While it encourages high standards, it can also lead to procrastination as individuals wait for the perfect conditions to begin a task.

Lack of Clarity:

Uncertainty about how to approach a task or where to start can cause individuals to procrastinate, as they feel overwhelmed and unsure of their abilities.

Instant Gratification:

The allure of immediate rewards, such as social media or entertainment, can distract individuals from their long-term goals, leading to procrastination.

Practical Strategies to Overcome Procrastination

1. Break Tasks into Smaller Steps:

Divide large tasks into smaller, more manageable steps. This makes them less intimidating and easier to tackle.

2. Set Clear Deadlines:

Establish deadlines for each task and hold yourself accountable to them. Use timers or calendar reminders to stay on track.

3. Use the Two-Minute Rule:

If a task takes less than two minutes to complete, do it immediately. This prevents small tasks from accumulating and becoming overwhelming.

4. Practice the "Five-Minute Rule":

Commit to working on a task for just five minutes. Often, getting started is the hardest part, and once you overcome that initial hurdle, momentum builds, making it easier to continue.

5. Create a Productive Environment:
Minimize distractions in your workspace by turning off notifications, decluttering your desk, and using tools like website blockers to limit access to distracting websites.

6. Use Positive Reinforcement:
Reward yourself for completing tasks or making progress towards your goals. Celebrate your accomplishments, no matter how small, to reinforce positive behavior.

7. Practice Self-Compassion:
Be kind to yourself when facing setbacks or challenges. Understand that everyone procrastinates occasionally, and it's okay to make mistakes. Focus on progress rather than perfection.

8. Visualize Success:
Imagine yourself completing the task successfully and experiencing the sense of accomplishment that comes with it. Visualization can increase motivation and reduce procrastination.

Maintaining Motivation and Momentum
Overcoming procrastination is an ongoing process that requires consistent effort and self-awareness. To maintain motivation and momentum, consider the following tips:

1. Set Clear Goals:
Clearly define your short-term and long-term goals to provide direction and purpose. Having a clear vision of what you want to achieve can keep you motivated and focused.

2. Establish a Routine:
Create a daily routine that includes dedicated time for work, relaxation, and self-care. Consistency helps build momentum and reduces the likelihood of procrastination.

3. Track Your Progress:
Keep track of your accomplishments and progress towards your goals. Celebrate your successes and use them as motivation to keep moving forward.

4. Stay Accountable:
Share your goals with a friend, family member, or mentor who can help hold you accountable. Regular check-ins can help you stay on track and avoid procrastination.

5. Reflect and Adjust:

Regularly reflect on your habits and behaviors to identify patterns of procrastination. Adjust your strategies as needed to overcome challenges and maintain momentum.

Conclusion

Procrastination is a common obstacle to effective time management and productivity, but it can be overcome with the right strategies and mindset. By understanding the root causes of procrastination and implementing practical techniques to address them, you can increase your productivity, reduce stress, and achieve your goals more effectively. Remember that overcoming procrastination is a journey, and with persistence and self-awareness, you can cultivate habits that lead to greater success and fulfillment.

Chapter 5: Creating a Productive Environment

Your environment plays a significant role in influencing your productivity and ability to focus. This chapter explores strategies for optimizing your physical and digital spaces to minimize distractions, enhance concentration, and create an environment conducive to productivity.

The Importance of Your Environment

Your environment encompasses both your physical surroundings, such as your workspace, and your digital environment, including your devices and online presence. A well-designed environment can boost your mood, increase motivation, and improve your ability to stay focused on tasks.

Physical Environment:

A clutter-free workspace reduces visual distractions and promotes mental clarity.

Ergonomic furniture and equipment minimize discomfort and enhance productivity.

Natural light and greenery can improve mood and creativity.

Digital Environment:

Organized digital files and folders make it easier to find information and stay focused on tasks.

Customized device settings, such as notification controls and screen time limits, help minimize distractions.

Utilizing productivity apps and tools can streamline workflows and keep tasks organized.

Tips for Creating a Productive Workspace

1. Declutter Your Space:

Remove unnecessary items from your workspace to reduce visual clutter and create a clean, organized environment.

2. Designate Specific Areas for Different Activities:
Create separate zones for work, relaxation, and leisure to establish boundaries and promote focus.

3. Personalize Your Space:
Surround yourself with items that inspire and motivate you, such as photos, artwork, or quotes.

4. Invest in Ergonomic Furniture:
Choose furniture that supports good posture and comfort to prevent physical discomfort and fatigue.

5. Optimize Lighting and Ventilation:
Ensure your workspace is well-lit and properly ventilated to promote alertness and concentration.

6. Minimize Distractions:
Identify and eliminate potential distractions, such as noisy appliances or tempting snacks, to maintain focus.

Organizing Your Digital Space

1. Digital Decluttering:
Regularly clean up your digital files, delete unnecessary emails, and uninstall unused apps to streamline your digital space.

2. Implement Folder Structures:
Create organized folder structures for storing digital files and documents, making it easier to locate information when needed.

3. Utilize Productivity Tools:
Take advantage of productivity apps and tools to manage tasks, schedule reminders, and track progress effectively.

4. Customize Device Settings:
Adjust notification settings, screen brightness, and other preferences to minimize distractions and optimize productivity.

Creating a Digital Detox Plan
While technology can enhance productivity, excessive digital consumption can lead to burnout and reduced focus. Incorporating regular digital detox sessions into your routine can help refresh your mind and prevent digital overload.

Digital Detox Strategies:
Designate specific times during the day for disconnecting from digital devices.

Engage in offline activities, such as reading, exercising, or spending time in nature.

Practice mindfulness techniques, such as meditation or deep breathing exercises, to reduce stress and promote relaxation.

Conclusion

Creating a productive environment involves optimizing both your physical and digital spaces to minimize distractions, foster concentration, and enhance productivity. By implementing strategies such as decluttering, personalizing your workspace, and organizing your digital files, you can create an environment that supports your goals and facilitates focus. Additionally, incorporating regular digital detox sessions into your routine can help prevent burnout and maintain a healthy work-life balance. With a well-designed environment, you can maximize your productivity and achieve your full potential.

Chapter 6: Utilizing Technology

In today's digital age, technology plays a crucial role in helping us manage our time and increase productivity. This chapter explores various technological tools and applications that can streamline your workflow, improve organization, and enhance efficiency.

Productivity Apps and Tools

Task Management Apps:

Trello: Trello is a popular project management tool that uses boards, lists, and cards to organize tasks and collaborate with team members. It's highly customizable and suitable for both personal and professional use.

Todoist: Todoist is a simple yet powerful task management app that allows you to create and prioritize tasks, set deadlines, and track your progress. It's available across multiple platforms and syncs seamlessly between devices.

Calendar Apps:

Google Calendar: Google Calendar is a widely used calendar app that enables you to schedule events, set reminders, and share calendars with others. Its intuitive interface and integration with other Google services make it a versatile tool for time management.

Apple Calendar: Apple Calendar, also known as iCal, is the default calendar app for Apple devices. It offers similar features to Google Calendar, including event scheduling, reminders, and calendar sharing.

Note-Taking Apps:
Evernote: Evernote is a comprehensive note-taking app that allows you to capture ideas, organize notes into notebooks, and sync across devices. It's ideal for brainstorming, project planning, and keeping track of information.
Microsoft OneNote: OneNote is a digital notebook that lets you create and organize notes, drawings, and audio recordings. It offers features like handwriting recognition, tag-based organization, and seamless integration with other Microsoft Office apps.

Balancing Technology Use
While technology can be a powerful tool for productivity, it's essential to strike a balance and avoid becoming overwhelmed or distracted by digital devices. Here are some strategies for maintaining a healthy relationship with technology:

Set Boundaries:
Establish designated times for using technology, such as checking emails or browsing social media. Limit screen time outside of these designated periods to prevent digital overload.

Use Technology Mindfully:
Be intentional about how you use technology. Instead of mindlessly scrolling through social media, use apps and tools that align with your goals and priorities.

Minimize Distractions:
Adjust your device settings to minimize distractions, such as turning off notifications or using focus modes that block access to distracting websites or apps during work sessions.

Leveraging Digital Tools for Time Management

Time Tracking Apps:
RescueTime: RescueTime is a time tracking app that monitors your digital activity and provides insights into how you spend your time online. It helps you identify time-wasting habits and optimize your productivity.
Toggl: Toggl is a simple time tracking app that allows you to track time spent on different tasks and projects. It's ideal for freelancers, consultants, and anyone who needs to bill clients based on hours worked.

Focus Apps:
Forest: Forest is a unique focus app that encourages you to stay focused by planting virtual trees. As you work without distractions,

your tree grows, but if you leave the app to check your phone, the tree dies. It's a fun and engaging way to boost productivity and minimize distractions.

Focus@Will: Focus@Will is a productivity app that uses neuroscience-based music playlists to help you concentrate and maintain focus. It offers a variety of music genres tailored to different work styles and preferences.

Integrating Technology into Your Workflow

To maximize the benefits of technology for productivity, consider integrating digital tools into your workflow in the following ways:

Streamline Communication:

Use communication tools like Slack or Microsoft Teams to collaborate with colleagues, share files, and stay connected in real-time.

Automate Repetitive Tasks:

Take advantage of automation tools like Zapier or IFTTT to automate repetitive tasks, such as sending email reminders, updating spreadsheets, or posting on social media.

Sync Across Devices:

Choose apps and tools that offer cross-platform compatibility and sync data across multiple devices. This ensures that you have access to your information whenever and wherever you need it.

Conclusion

Technology offers a wealth of opportunities for enhancing productivity and managing time more effectively. By leveraging productivity apps, balancing technology use, and integrating digital tools into your workflow, you can streamline your tasks, minimize distractions, and focus on what truly matters. However, it's essential to use technology mindfully and establish healthy boundaries to prevent digital overload and maintain work-life balance. With the right approach, technology can be a valuable ally in your quest for greater productivity and success.

Chapter 7: Building Healthy Habits for Long-Term Success

Building and maintaining healthy habits is essential for long-term productivity and overall well-being. This chapter explores the science behind habit formation, strategies for cultivating positive habits, and techniques for sustaining them over time.

Understanding Habit Formation

Habits are automatic behaviors that are triggered by cues in your environment and reinforced by rewards. They are formed through a process called habit loop, which consists of three stages:

Cue: The trigger that prompts the behavior. It could be a specific time of day, a particular location, or an emotional state.

Routine: The behavior itself, which is the habitual response to the cue.

Reward: The positive reinforcement that reinforces the behavior and increases the likelihood of it recurring in the future.

Understanding the habit loop allows you to identify patterns in your behavior and develop strategies for creating and changing habits effectively.

Strategies for Cultivating Positive Habits

1. Start Small:

Begin by focusing on small, manageable habits that are easy to incorporate into your daily routine. Gradually increase the complexity and difficulty of the habits over time.

2. Set Clear Goals:

Define specific, measurable goals for each habit you want to develop. Having clear objectives provides direction and motivation.

3. Create Implementation Intentions:

Formulate if-then statements that link the desired habit to a specific cue and response. For example, "If it's 6:00 AM, then I will go for a morning run."

4. Use Habit Stacking:

Anchor new habits to existing routines or behaviors to leverage existing cues and increase the likelihood of adoption. For instance, "After brushing my teeth, I will meditate for five minutes."

5. Monitor Progress:

Keep track of your habit implementation using habit tracking apps or simple journaling techniques. Monitoring progress allows you to identify areas for improvement and celebrate successes.

Techniques for Sustaining Habits

1. Practice Consistency:

Make a commitment to consistently perform the desired behavior, even on days when motivation is low. Consistency is key to solidifying habits over time.

2. Embrace Imperfection:

Accept that occasional setbacks or lapses are a normal part of the habit-building process. Instead of dwelling on failures, focus on getting back on track and learning from your experiences.

3. Use Reinforcement:

Reward yourself for sticking to your habits and achieving milestones along the way. Positive reinforcement reinforces the behavior and increases its likelihood of becoming ingrained.

4. Cultivate a Growth Mindset:

Adopt a growth mindset that views challenges and setbacks as opportunities for learning and growth. Embrace the journey of habit formation as a process of self-improvement and personal development.

Incorporating Self-Care into Your Routine

In addition to productivity-related habits, it's essential to prioritize self-care habits that support your physical, mental, and emotional well-being. Examples of self-care habits include:

Getting an adequate amount of sleep each night.

Engaging in regular exercise and physical activity.

Practicing mindfulness or meditation to reduce stress.

Nourishing your body with nutritious foods and staying hydrated.

Carving out time for hobbies, relaxation, and leisure activities.

Conclusion

Building healthy habits is a foundational component of long-term success and well-being. By understanding the science of habit formation and implementing strategies for cultivating and sustaining positive habits, you can make meaningful changes to your life. Whether you're striving to improve productivity, enhance your health, or foster personal growth, developing healthy habits empowers you to live a more fulfilling and purposeful life. Remember that building habits is a gradual process that requires patience, persistence, and self-awareness. With dedication and commitment, you can transform your habits and unlock your full potential.

Chapter 8: Effective Stress Management Strategies

Stress is a common part of life, but when left unmanaged, it can negatively impact your physical health, mental well-being, and overall productivity. This chapter explores the causes and effects of stress, as well as practical strategies for managing stress effectively.

Understanding Stress

Stress is your body's natural response to perceived threats or challenges. While some level of stress can be beneficial, chronic or excessive stress can lead to a range of negative consequences, including:

Physical Effects: Headaches, muscle tension, fatigue, and digestive issues.

Mental Effects: Anxiety, irritability, difficulty concentrating, and mood swings.

Behavioral Effects: Changes in appetite, sleep disturbances, and withdrawal from social activities.

Long-Term Health Risks: Chronic stress has been linked to an increased risk of cardiovascular disease, obesity, diabetes, and other serious health conditions.

Identifying Sources of Stress

To effectively manage stress, it's essential to identify the specific sources or triggers of stress in your life. Common sources of stress include:

Work-related Stress : Tight deadlines, heavy workloads, conflicts with colleagues, or job insecurity.

Personal Relationships: Conflict with family members, friends, or romantic partners.

Financial Pressures : Debt, unemployment, or financial instability.

Health Concerns: Chronic illnesses, injuries, or health-related anxieties.

Life Transitions: Major life changes such as moving, divorce, marriage, or parenthood.

Practical Stress Management Strategies

1. Practice Relaxation Techniques:

Incorporate relaxation techniques such as deep breathing, meditation, progressive muscle relaxation, or guided imagery into your daily routine to reduce stress levels and promote relaxation.

2. Prioritize Self-Care:

Make self-care a priority by engaging in activities that nourish your body, mind, and soul. This includes getting adequate sleep, eating a balanced diet, exercising regularly, and setting aside time for hobbies and leisure activities.

3. Maintain a Healthy Lifestyle:

Adopt healthy lifestyle habits that support overall well-being, such as regular exercise, nutritious eating, limiting caffeine and alcohol intake, and avoiding tobacco use.

4. Set Boundaries:

Establish clear boundaries to protect your time, energy, and emotional well-being. Learn to say no to commitments or requests that overwhelm or drain you.

5. Practice Time Management:

Use effective time management techniques to prioritize tasks, set realistic goals, and allocate time for important activities. This helps reduce feelings of overwhelm and improves productivity.

6. Seek Social Support:

Reach out to friends, family members, or support groups for emotional support and encouragement. Talking to others about your stressors can provide perspective and help alleviate feelings of isolation.

7. Engage in Stress-Relieving Activities:

Participate in activities that promote relaxation and stress relief, such as spending time in nature, listening to music, practicing yoga or tai chi, or enjoying a hot bath.

8. Seek Professional Help:

If stress becomes overwhelming or significantly impacts your daily functioning, consider seeking support from a mental health professional. Therapy, counseling, or stress management programs can provide additional tools and strategies for coping with stress.

Conclusion

Effective stress management is essential for maintaining overall health, well-being, and productivity. By understanding the sources of stress in your life and implementing practical strategies for stress reduction, you can minimize its negative effects and improve your quality of life. Remember that managing stress is an ongoing process that requires self-awareness, resilience, and a commitment to self-care. By prioritizing your physical, mental, and emotional well-being, you can build resilience to stress and thrive in the face of life's challenges.

Chapter 9: Enhancing Focus and Concentration

In today's fast-paced world full of distractions, maintaining focus and concentration is essential for productivity and success. This chapter explores the importance of focus, common challenges to concentration, and practical strategies for enhancing your ability to stay focused on tasks.

The Importance of Focus

Focus is the ability to direct your attention and concentration toward a specific task or goal while ignoring distractions. It allows you to work efficiently, solve problems effectively, and achieve your objectives. However, in an age of constant connectivity and information overload, maintaining focus has become increasingly challenging.

Common Challenges to Concentration

Several factors can undermine your ability to focus and concentrate, including:

Digital Distractions: Constant notifications, emails, and social media updates can disrupt your train of thought and divert your attention away from important tasks.

Multitasking: Trying to juggle multiple tasks simultaneously can lead to decreased productivity and reduced effectiveness in completing each task.

Physical Discomfort: Uncomfortable work environments, such as noise, temperature extremes, or uncomfortable seating, can make it difficult to concentrate for extended periods.

Mental Fatigue: Prolonged periods of cognitive effort or decision-making can lead to mental fatigue, diminishing your ability to maintain focus and concentration.

Strategies for Enhancing Focus and Concentration

1. Minimize Distractions:

Create a distraction-free work environment by turning off notifications, closing unnecessary tabs or applications, and finding a quiet space to work.

2. Practice Mindfulness:

Incorporate mindfulness techniques, such as meditation or deep breathing exercises, into your daily routine to improve focus, reduce stress, and increase awareness of the present moment.

3. Break Tasks into Manageable Segments:

Divide large tasks into smaller, more manageable segments, and focus on completing one segment at a time. This prevents feelings of overwhelm and helps maintain focus.

4. Use Time Blocking:

Allocate dedicated time blocks for specific tasks or activities, and focus exclusively on those tasks during each block. This helps minimize distractions and increase productivity.

5. Set Clear Goals and Priorities:
Define specific, achievable goals for each task, and prioritize them based on importance and urgency. Having clear objectives provides direction and motivation, making it easier to stay focused.

6. Take Regular Breaks:
Schedule short breaks throughout your workday to rest and recharge. Taking breaks can help prevent mental fatigue and maintain focus and productivity over time.

7. Practice the Pomodoro Technique:
Use the Pomodoro Technique to break your work into short, focused intervals (typically 25 minutes) followed by brief breaks. This helps maintain concentration and prevent burnout.

8. Exercise Regularly:
Engage in regular physical activity, as exercise has been shown to improve cognitive function, memory, and focus.

9. Get Adequate Sleep:
Prioritize sleep and aim for 7-9 hours of quality sleep each night. Sleep deprivation can impair cognitive function and diminish your ability to concentrate.

Conclusion
Enhancing focus and concentration is a skill that can be developed and improved with practice. By implementing strategies such as minimizing distractions, practicing mindfulness, breaking tasks into manageable segments, and prioritizing self-care, you can strengthen your ability to maintain focus and productivity in all areas of your life. Remember that building focus is a gradual process that requires patience, consistency, and self-awareness. With dedication and effort, you can sharpen your focus and achieve greater success in your personal and professional endeavors.

Chapter 10: Effective Communication Skills
Effective communication is essential for building strong relationships, fostering collaboration, and achieving success in both personal and professional settings. This chapter explores the key components of effective communication, common barriers to communication, and strategies for improving your communication skills.

The Importance of Effective Communication

Communication is the process of exchanging information, ideas, and feelings between individuals or groups. Effective communication enhances clarity, understanding, and connection, while poor communication can lead to misunderstandings, conflict, and inefficiency.

Key Components of Effective Communication

1. Clear and Concise Messaging:

Communicate your message clearly and concisely, using simple language and avoiding jargon or unnecessary complexity.

2. Active Listening:

Practice active listening by giving your full attention to the speaker, maintaining eye contact, and providing feedback to demonstrate understanding.

3. Empathy and Understanding:

Show empathy and understanding towards others' perspectives, feelings, and experiences, even if you disagree with them.

4. Nonverbal Communication:

Pay attention to nonverbal cues such as facial expressions, body language, and tone of voice, as they often convey more meaning than words alone.

5. Assertiveness:

Express your thoughts, opinions, and needs clearly and respectfully, while also being open to feedback and differing viewpoints.

Common Barriers to Communication

1. Poor Listening Skills:

Inattentiveness, interrupting, or preoccupation with one's thoughts can hinder effective listening and understanding.

2. Assumptions and Stereotypes:

Making assumptions or relying on stereotypes about others can lead to misinterpretation and misunderstanding.

3. Emotional Reactions:

Strong emotions such as anger, frustration, or anxiety can impair communication by clouding judgment and triggering defensive responses.

4. Language Barriers:

Differences in language or cultural norms can create barriers to communication, requiring sensitivity and adaptability to overcome.

Strategies for Improving Communication Skills

1. Practice Active Listening:
Focus on fully understanding the speaker's message before
formulating your response. Ask clarifying questions and paraphrase
to ensure mutual understanding.
2. Be Clear and Specific:
Use clear and specific language to convey your message, avoiding
vague or ambiguous terms that can lead to confusion.
3. Seek Feedback:
Solicit feedback from others on your communication style and
actively incorporate constructive criticism to improve your skills.
4. Cultivate Empathy:
Put yourself in the other person's shoes and consider their
perspective and feelings when communicating. Empathy fosters
understanding and connection.
5. Practice Assertiveness:
Assert yourself respectfully and confidently, expressing your
thoughts and needs while also listening to and respecting others'
perspectives.
6. Manage Emotions Effectively:
Learn to recognize and regulate your emotions during
communication to prevent emotional reactions from interfering with
clarity and understanding.
7. Adapt to Your Audience:
Tailor your communication style to suit the preferences and needs of
your audience, whether it be colleagues, clients, friends, or family
members.

Conclusion

Effective communication is a fundamental skill that contributes to
success in all aspects of life. By mastering the key components of
effective communication, identifying and addressing common
barriers, and practicing strategies for improvement, you can enhance
your ability to connect with others, build stronger relationships, and
achieve your goals. Remember that communication is a dynamic
process that requires ongoing effort, self-awareness, and practice.
With dedication and perseverance, you can become a more effective
communicator and unlock new opportunities for growth and success.

Chapter 11: Conflict Resolution Strategies

Conflict is a natural part of human interaction, but when managed
effectively, it can lead to growth, innovation, and stronger

relationships. This chapter explores the nature of conflict, common sources of conflict, and strategies for resolving conflicts in constructive ways.

Understanding Conflict

Conflict arises when individuals or groups have differing interests, values, or perspectives, leading to tension, disagreement, or misunderstanding. While conflict is often viewed negatively, it can also present opportunities for learning, problem-solving, and relationship-building.

Common Sources of Conflict

1. Miscommunication:

Poor communication, misunderstandings, or ambiguous messages can create confusion and lead to conflict.

2. Differences in Values or Beliefs:

Divergent values, beliefs, or cultural norms can clash, resulting in conflict over how to approach certain issues or decisions.

3. Competition for Resources:

Scarce resources such as time, money, or opportunities can spark conflict as individuals or groups vie for access or control.

4. Personality Clashes:

Differences in personality, communication styles, or work habits can lead to interpersonal conflicts within teams or organizations.

Strategies for Conflict Resolution

1. Active Listening:

Listen attentively to the concerns and perspectives of all parties involved, demonstrating empathy and understanding.

2. Clarify Perceptions:

Encourage open dialogue to clarify misunderstandings, address assumptions, and gain insight into each other's perspectives.

3. Find Common Ground:

Identify shared goals or interests and work collaboratively to find mutually beneficial solutions that satisfy everyone involved.

4. Focus on Interests, Not Positions:

Look beyond surface-level demands or positions to understand the underlying interests or needs driving each party's stance.

5. Explore Creative Solutions:

Brainstorm alternative solutions or compromises that address the interests of all parties and promote win-win outcomes.

6. Maintain Respect and Civility:

Foster a respectful and supportive atmosphere that values diverse opinions and encourages constructive dialogue.

7. Seek Mediation or Facilitation:

Engage a neutral third party to facilitate communication, mediate disputes, and help find resolution in complex or entrenched conflicts.

8. Practice Forgiveness and Letting Go:

Let go of grudges or resentments and focus on moving forward with a mindset of forgiveness and reconciliation.

Implementing Conflict Resolution Strategies

1. Establish Clear Communication Channels:

Create open lines of communication and provide opportunities for all parties to express their concerns and perspectives.

2. Develop Conflict Resolution Skills:

Invest in training or workshops to enhance conflict resolution skills among team members or organizational leaders.

3. Foster a Positive Organizational Culture:

Cultivate a culture that values transparency, collaboration, and constructive feedback, minimizing the likelihood of conflicts escalating.

4. Address Conflict Proactively:

Anticipate potential sources of conflict and address them proactively before they escalate into more significant issues.

Conclusion

Conflict resolution is a critical skill that enables individuals and organizations to navigate differences, overcome challenges, and foster positive relationships. By understanding the nature of conflict, identifying common sources of conflict, and implementing effective conflict resolution strategies, you can turn conflicts into opportunities for growth, innovation, and collaboration. Remember that conflict resolution is not about avoiding or suppressing disagreements but rather managing them constructively and finding solutions that benefit everyone involved. With patience, empathy, and a willingness to engage in open dialogue, you can resolve conflicts effectively and create a harmonious and productive environment for all.

Chapter 12: Conclusion: Embracing Growth and Gratitude

As we reach the conclusion of this book, it's essential to reflect on the journey we've taken together. Throughout these pages, we've explored a diverse range of topics aimed at enhancing motivation, productivity, and overall well-being. From understanding the psychology of motivation to mastering time management techniques, from fostering resilience to cultivating healthy habits, each chapter has offered valuable insights and practical strategies for personal and professional growth.

But beyond the strategies and techniques lies a deeper message: the power of gratitude. In our pursuit of success and self-improvement, it's easy to overlook the blessings and opportunities that surround us every day. Gratitude is the practice of acknowledging and appreciating the good in our lives, whether big or small. It shifts our focus from what we lack to what we have, from scarcity to abundance.

So as you embark on your journey towards a more motivated, productive, and fulfilling life, remember to cultivate an attitude of gratitude. Take a moment each day to reflect on the things you're thankful for, whether it's supportive relationships, meaningful work, or moments of joy and beauty. Embrace challenges as opportunities for growth, setbacks as lessons to be learned, and successes as milestones on your path to greatness.

I want to extend my heartfelt thanks to you, the reader, for joining me on this journey. Your curiosity, openness, and willingness to learn are what make this exploration possible. May the insights and strategies shared in these pages serve as guiding lights on your path to success and fulfillment.

With gratitude and best wishes,
Himanshi Dwivedi